Adrenal Fatigue

Take Control of Adrenal Burnout And Restore Your Health Naturally

Christine Weil

Christine Weil

Table of Contents

Introduction

I want to thank you and congratulate you for purchasing the book, "Adrenal Fatigue: Take Control of Adrenal Burnout and Restore Your Health Naturally".

This book contains valuable information and steps to treat Adrenal Fatigue, and recover your sense of wellbeing.

If you are reading this guide, then chances are either you or someone close to you is experiencing symptoms of adrenal fatigue. The information contained here will explain what adrenal fatigue is, how to tell if you have it, and how to treat it successfully. You will want to keep this guide handy for quick referrals, guidance, and tips for fighting adrenal fatigue.

Thank you again for purchasing this book; I hope you enjoy it!

Christine Weil

What is Adrenal Fatigue?

Adrenal fatigue is a set of physical symptoms that is the result of decreased function of the adrenal glands. Symptoms include, but are not limited to, fatigue not relieved by adequate sleep, need for the use of stimulants (caffeine, nicotine), and a general feeling of ill health. Though not considered a medical diagnosis, it is believed that a great majority of Americans have experienced some form of this disease at some point in their lives. Traditional medicine recognizes only the extreme forms of adrenal dysfunction, known as adrenal insufficiency. Those who suffer from adrenal fatigue do not experience the degree of illness seen with the more critical diagnosis, but they do feel a decrease in the quality of their life. To understand the mechanism of adrenal fatigue and how it affects the individual in the way that it does, it is best to describe the function of the adrenal glands.

The adrenal glands are small, triangle-shaped glands located on the top surface of both kidneys. They help regulate blood pressure, blood sugar levels, sodium and potassium balance, and the stress response. They do this through the production of hormones, such as aldosterone (sodium regulation), cortisol (stress response), and adrenaline and noradrenaline – the hormones that are involved in the "fight or flight" response. The output of these hormones is regulated by feedback signals from the brain. For example, the eyes sense danger, say an oncoming car, and send a message to the adrenals to secrete adrenaline and cortisol. These hormones allow us to remove ourselves from harm's way by heightening our sensitivity, and giving us that extra boost of energy needed. After the danger has passed, the body returns to a normal state, and the adrenals stop secreting the level of hormones needed to sustain this response.

In non-threatening situations, there are relatively low levels of these hormones being produced. There are only enough in circulation to maintain normal body functioning. However, in times of severe stress, the adrenal gland receives feedback from the brain that the body is in ongoing danger. This causes the adrenals to continually release these hormones. This constant overproduction depletes the glands of these substances, and leads to "burn out" of the adrenal glands, and a state of adrenal fatigue. Adrenal fatigue is not to be confused with adrenal insufficiency, which is a more severe form adrenal gland dysfunction. It requires lifelong treatment by a medical provider, and the use of steroids to prevent a dangerous health crisis. Fortunately, the effects of adrenal fatigue can be treated without the use of medications. The individual can usually maintain her adrenal health in more natural ways. The focus of this book will be to inform you about what symptoms to look for if you suspect adrenal fatigue, and what natural ways of healing the condition and preventing its recurrence are available to you.

Signs and Symptoms of Adrenal Fatigue

Now that you have been introduced to the syndrome of adrenal fatigue, you are probably curious as to how it presents. Actually, many disease states can mimic adrenal fatigue. It is prudent to check with your health care professional to check for other medical conditions that may require different forms of therapy. However, once these conditions have been ruled out, adrenal fatigue should be seriously considered. Below is a list of common symptoms that are associated with adrenal "burnout":

- Sleep disturbances (insomnia)
- Cravings for salty or sweet foods
- Increased need for stimulants (caffeine, nicotine)
- Low blood pressure
- Decreased body hair
- Prolonged recuperation from illnesses
- General body aches/pains
- Having more energy in the afternoon than morning
- Difficulty getting out of bed after a good night's sleep
- Increase in severity of PMS/menopause symptoms
- Weight loss (without trying)
- Feeling "overwhelmed" by life
- Unstable behavior/mood swings
- Memory/Concentration problems
- Inflammation
- Gastric disturbances (indigestion, bloating)
- Exhausted after a normal workout
- Dark under-eye circles

Other, lesser known symptoms include:

- Dependence on sunglasses (increased sensitivity to sunlight)
- Hollow cheeks (not related to a known medical condition)
- Verticals lines in fingertip pads
- Pale lips (in absence of anemia)
- Increased allergies
- Lower sex drive
- Prone to infections
- Depression
- Inability to handle stress – "high strung"
- Auto immune problems

As you can see, the list includes symptoms which can mimic many other diseases. For example, clinical depression can produce a number of these signs, especially those related to sleep disturbances and mood swings. Hormonal imbalances, drug interactions, vitamin deficiencies, pregnancy, chronic fatigue syndrome, cancer, and diabetes should all be excluded with physical examinations and testing. However, in the absence of any of these conditions, adrenal fatigue should be taken into account. Treatment should be started to improve the well-being of the person experiencing this distress.

What are the Causes?

The list of causes of adrenal fatigue can be as numerous and varied as the list of symptoms. In a nutshell, any situation that provokes a severe and sustained stress response can lead to adrenal fatigue. This can be anything from an acute trauma to a prolonged state of constant tension. Below you will find a list of the most common scenarios:

- Major illness or infection (especially respiratory)
- Exposure to environmental toxins
- Malnutrition
- Major surgery
- Drug/alcohol addiction
- Major physical trauma (amputation, injury to vital organs)
- Psychological trauma (rape, assault, abuse)
- Emotional stress (relationship issues, harassment)
- Financial problems
- Employment difficulties
- Overuse of stimulants
- Sleep deprivation
- Constant physical/mental stress (perpetual "fight or flight" status)
- Unexpected loss of people or property
- Poor diet/eating habits
- Zinc deficiency
- Lack of self-care
- Lack of a support system

As you can see, there are many situations that can propel us into a state of constant stress, and lead to the decreased function of our adrenal glands. There are some triggers that are uncommon and fortunately, most of us will not experience those. Situations such as a suffering a major health crisis, witnessing the devastation of a natural disaster, or surviving an extremely traumatic event, can carry additional complications that require immediate attention, and can mask the presence of adrenal fatigue. Severe malnutrition and major surgery are also less common, but important causes.

However, almost everyone alive in this day and age will be exposed to some level of stress, sometimes very high levels, for a brief period of time. Letting it go unchecked or unacknowledged could lead to adrenal fatigue. Our poor Western diet and haphazard eating habits are, not surprisingly, a major contributor to this condition, and go hand-in-hand with a lack of self-care and exposure to toxins or unhealthy substances in our food. Zinc deficiency has recently been linked to adrenal fatigue. It was found that individuals who received zinc supplements had a decrease in the severity of symptoms over time. This is an exciting find that hopefully will justify further research.

Who is Susceptible?

Anyone living in the world today can be susceptible to adrenal fatigue. With a society that demands instant gratification, applies constant pressure to perform, has financial instability, political uncertainty, and an increase in violence worldwide, we are continuously exposed to a culture of fear. Although no formal studies have been performed, it has been estimated that as many as 66% of the population has experienced adrenal fatigue at one point and 16% could be classified as having severe cases. These numbers are not surprising and are most likely on the rise. In addition to the factors previously mentioned, we are also a society that has become increasingly isolated from each other. Systems of family and community support for the individual are weakening, and we've become more and more dependent on technology for communication. This lack of physical interaction can increase the level of stress, since it does not allow for the positive feedback that takes place in a supportive environment.

As for gender, adrenal fatigue appears to effect men and women equally, although women are more likely to seek help when they feel unwell, especially if there is no obvious symptom to report. Also, women tend to be the caretakers in many circumstances, and will often sacrifice their own health and comfort for the sake of others. The stress of a new mother, or of an adult child caring for an elderly parent, or of a spouse caring for a disabled partner, are all situations that produce a large amount of ongoing tension that can make a person more vulnerable to adrenal fatigue. As for men, the pressure to maintain a certain level of financial success, and to constantly perform at "the top of their game" can most definitely cause over exposure to high stress levels. With all of the distractions of the modern age, the time to refresh ourselves is limited. And also frowned upon in a society where rest = weakness. Considering all of these issues, it is a wonder that adrenal fatigue is not present in 100% of the adult population!

People who struggle with relationship issues are more susceptible to adrenal fatigue. Not only have we seen a decrease in more personal forms of communication, stress from other areas of life can trickle into personal relationships and cause complications. Feelings of inadequacy, anxiety, and confusion over the state of a relationship can tax the adrenal glands as severely as other forms of stress. Toxic relationships with negative people can be especially damaging and could trigger the stress response as well.

The Effects of Nutrition and Lifestyle

If you look at the diet of the average American, it is a wonder we are not worse off than we are. We have become a nation of fast food addicts, hopped up on caffeine with a constant sugar high, and with very little in the way of regular exercise. Obviously this does not pertain to everyone, but we do like our fat and salt, and our quality time with Judge Judy.

Even for those of us who resist taking up permanent residence at McDonald's, there is still the common habit of skipping meals. Erratic mealtimes can do a number on the adrenal glands as it becomes more difficult to maintain a constant blood sugar level with normal amounts of hormones, cortisol in particular.

When a person skips a meal or drags out time between meals for too long, they tend to eat large amounts of the "wrong" types of foods, such as carbohydrates and high fat products. This causes the glands to secrete greater amounts of hormone to deal with the drastic increase in blood sugar. After this has happened, there is a sudden decrease in cortisol levels, as the adrenals have had to produce a higher than normal level to deal with all of that sugar. This can lead to the extreme energy low that is experienced after one of these episodes, which inevitably leads to the use/abuse of stimulants to maintain the energy needed to complete the day.

Adrenal hormones are also over-produced in the presence of caffeine and other stimulants. These substances act like the fight or flight response to "kick start" the adrenals to release adrenaline to give the individual a boost of energy. Elimination of these products will go a long way in restoring the adrenal glands to their normal state. Ironically, the more pronounced the adrenal fatigue is, the more the sufferer increases their intake to combat the symptoms of sleepiness and lack of energy.

You can probably see the vicious cycle that is going on here. A person eats a large meal full of fat/carbohydrates, crashes an hour later (usually in the afternoon when there is still work to be done), then takes a large amount of caffeine to get a second wind, and continues the unrelenting assault on the adrenal glands. This leads to adrenal fatigue, which worsens the symptoms, causing the individual to consume foods high in salt or sugar, which leads to extreme energy lows, which they then treat with caffeine. So you can see how hard it is to break the cycle once it reaches this point.

Another thing to consider is the presence of additional hormones in our food supply. Even if you don't indulge in fast food, some of the food found in the local market can contain substances that affect the adrenals. For many years, it was common practice to give livestock hormones to increase milk supply (in the case of cows), or produce larger animals to feed more people. This is one case where bigger definitely wasn't better.

Consuming unknown amounts of hormones in our diet can disrupt the hormonal balance in our own bodies. The adrenal glands are sensitive to changes in hormonal concentrations, even small ones, and will adjust to maintain a normal state. If they are being constantly bombarded with these substances, they become overworked. This can be avoided by looking for meat that does not contain hormones and is raised in a more natural environment.

Lifestyle practices that can affect the function of the adrenal glands are numerous. We have previously discussed the presence of constant stress and exposure to negativity as making someone more vulnerable to adrenal fatigue. Lack of regular exercise can also be a factor. Exercise gives a natural boost of energy that can aid in the normal production of adrenal hormones, such as cortisol and adrenaline, and maintain a state of well-being. Most Americans have a rather sedentary lifestyle, which can be both cause and/or effect of our poor diet. Not engaging in regular exercise actually decreases your energy level, and can increase the dependence on stimulants for an energy boost.

Another culprit is lack of adequate sleep. The body requires a certain amount of rest to recuperate from its daily activities. With so many distractions and the pressure to constantly be "productive," sleep has become a luxury for many. However, denying the body this period of relaxation causes it to be fatigued, which leads to - you guessed it - stress. The adrenals respond appropriately, but if this is an ongoing issue, they will eventually start to burn out, and the symptoms of adrenal fatigue will appear.

The Traditional Medicine Approach to Adrenal Fatigue

Adrenal fatigue is not a recognized diagnosis in the traditional medical community. Currently only the more extreme form of malfunction, adrenal insufficiency, or Addison's disease, is acknowledged. This is not to say that it is not a real entity. In fact, some physicians do believe that the condition exists, and that it can impact the health of the individual who suffers from the symptoms. However, the vast majority do not believe that it should be considered a true diagnosis, and they cite a lack of compelling scientific evidence to prove their point.

The stance of the modern medical community is understandable to a certain extent. Modern medicine has become more dependent on diagnostic tests to look for abnormalities. In the past, these tests were used to complement the history and physical exam in determining the presence of disease in the patient. Now, they are used in place of the more personal methods. This is largely due to the more scientific model of medicine; if there is not enough laboratory data to support the presence of a certain condition, then it is not the cause of the ailment.

In the case of adrenal insufficiency, there is a pronounced decrease in the amount of hormones (namely cortisol) detected, therefore supporting the physical diagnosis of the disease. However, with adrenal fatigue, levels of hormones may appear to be low-normal to normal in most people. Individuals respond differently to hormonal changes, some being more sensitive than others. Current traditional methods of testing are inadequate for detecting the subtle changes in hormones, but they are still considered standard in traditional medicine and as such do not support a diagnosis of adrenal fatigue.

The other argument used in traditional medicine is that the symptoms can be caused by other medically accepted disease states. Physicians caution against using an unsupported diagnosis and somehow missing the correct one. Fortunately, most of these other conditions have reliable methods of testing, so if the results are normal, then it is likely that they are not the cause. However, historically it has been the rule and not the exception for medicine to reverse its previous position once new information has been discovered. This has happened in many instances, most notably with conditions that had multiple symptoms and could not easily be tested. Examples are chronic fatigue syndrome, fibromyalgia, and depression, to name a few. With this in mind, it may only be a matter of time before traditional medicine accepts adrenal fatigue as a valid diagnosis.

How to Test for Adrenal Fatigue

Although we spent the last chapter bemoaning the inadequacy of testing for adrenal fatigue, it was in reference to the testing standards of *traditional* medicine. For alternative practitioners, there are tests available that can help you determine if you are affected by adrenal fatigue. The most common method is a saliva test. The saliva test is reported to be more sensitive than the blood test due to the more accurate detection of cortisol levels.

The belief is that one must not be stressed when being tested for cortisol levels. With a blood test, a patient must be stuck with a needle to collect a sample. The idea in and of itself is stressful to most people and the pain experienced could lead to an increase in cortisol levels, which could give a falsely elevated number. Although not the most sophisticated of methods, the saliva tests presents little in the way of stress and should not cause any additional increase in cortisol, allowing for a more accurate reading.

Saliva testing does not require the approval of a physician and can be done at home using any of the commercially available tests (ZRT and Genova labs provide these tests directly to the individual). However, you should locate a health professional who will agree to interpret the findings for you. For the most precise results, the samples are taken 4 times a day according to the instructions provided. Based on the levels found, the practitioner could determine a treatment regimen to improve the symptoms of adrenal fatigue and reverse it entirely.

In spite of all of this talk of tests and hormone levels, the most valuable way to determine the presence of adrenal fatigue is to examine the individual. Getting a history that describes the symptoms and when they occurred can lead your provider toward a proper diagnosis and allow you to undergo treatment sooner.

Remember, you are ultimately responsible for the way you feel; if you think that something is wrong, then search for the cause and get additional opinions. Be sure and answer questions honestly and as accurately as possible. This will enable the provider to get the information needed to successfully treat your condition.

Christine Weil

Natural Treatments

Now it's time for the good news. You've read about adrenal fatigue, what causes it, what symptoms are present, how common it is, and how to diagnose. Ok, now that you know you have it, what do you do? Well, hopefully you will get treated for it and start taking your life back. Many of the symptoms of adrenal fatigue can be reversed by simply removing the causes. First, you may want to look at your diet and eating habits and see if this is where the problem lies. The next chapter will give recipe ideas for adrenal fatigue, but these suggestions should give you a good starting point for recovery and improve your health in other areas, too. Diet changes that will improve your symptoms include:

Schedule regular meal times – Avoid skipping meals, and then gorging later in the day. This will maintain normal blood sugar levels and take the pressure off the adrenals.

Avoiding sugar/processed foods – Large quantities of sugar cause a sudden drop in energy and increase the work of the adrenals. Less is more...

Eliminate stimulants – This can be very difficult for folks who require the 12 steps to get off caffeine, but it is worth it, and your adrenals will thank you. A healthy alternative is green tea.

Increase vegetable/protein intake – This will give your body the fuel it needs and eliminate the amount of waste. Your adrenals AND your intestines will thank you.

Increase the intake of "good" fats – Foods like avocados, nuts, and coconut oil will provide a more stable source of energy and prevent the highs and lows associated with sugars.
Increase the intake of "good" salt – Not all salt is bad for you. In fact, you need the presence of good salt, like

20

Himalayan crystal salt, to aid the function of the adrenal glands.

Drink lots of water – I know it seems like the answer to everything, but dehydration can cause stress and cause you to overeat, both of which cause the adrenals to work harder and burn out sooner.

Other natural treatments include taking dietary supplements like zinc (which was mentioned previously), B complex vitamins, Niacin, and DHEA to name a few.

- Niacin, or vitamin B3, helps balance hormones, increases cortisol production, and prevents adrenal damage.
- B complex vitamins can help improve adrenal function as they help eliminate toxins and regulate stress hormones.
- Zinc, one of the newest discoveries, has been found to calm the nervous system and increase energy levels.
- DHEA is the precursor to the sex hormones and can treat symptoms of adrenal fatigue by increasing energy levels, a sense of well-being, and libido. However, using DHEA supplements in the absence of a deficiency can be harmful. Side effects for women can include increased estrogen production, which can lead to mood changes and sleep disturbances. In men, there is increased testosterone production, which can lead to hair loss and prostate irritation. It is highly recommended that you take the saliva test to check DHEA levels before starting any supplement.

For further information, consult your holistic provider for the correct dosages and frequency of any supplements you wish to take.

Recipes for Adrenal Fatigue

As promised, here are a few recipes that you can try that can help with your symptoms.

Black Bean Salad
Serves 4

1 (15-ounce) can black beans, drained, rinsed, and chilled
1 mango, diced
1/2 red bell pepper, diced
1 scallion, sliced thinly
2 tablespoons extra virgin olive oil
2 teaspoons red wine vinegar
1 to 2 teaspoons minced jalapeno
1/4 teaspoon dried cilantro
Salt to taste
2 tablespoons crumbled goat cheese

Mix everything but the cheese in a bowl. Allow to marinate in the refrigerator for an hour before serving for best flavor. Add cheese just before serving.

nutrition info per serving: 271 calories, 10 g fat, 3 g saturated fat, 7 mg cholesterol, 12 g protein, 35 g carbohydrates, 11 g fiber, 28 mg sodium

Lava Flow Hand Rolls With Onion-Soy Sauce
Serves 4

1/4 onion, diced
1/4 teaspoon rice wine vinegar
1/4 teaspoon lemon juice
4 tablespoons soy sauce
4 large leaves of red chard
3/4 cup cooked brown sushi rice
8 (1-ounce) slices of sushi-grade, raw ahi tuna
8 slices of ripe papaya, about the same size as the ahi slices
1 avocado, sliced into eighths
1 ounce of microgreens or sprouts, evenly divided for four rolls
4 roughly chopped macadamia nuts

1. Place onion, vinegar, lemon juice, and soy sauce in a small bowl, and set aside.

2. Lightly steam the chard leaves for 2 minutes. Run under cool water, and pat dry. Stack 2 leaves on top of each other with the underside up and the thick side of the stems closest to you. Fill the center with 2 to 3 tablespoons of rice, flush with the thick edge of the stem, leaving the upper half of the leaf empty.

3. Add 2 slices each of ahi, papaya, and avocado. Top with microgreens and one chopped macadamia, fold the sides together, and bring the bottom of the leaf up over them. Repeat with remaining chard leaves.

4. Spoon onion-soy mixture inside and serve.

nutrition info per serving: 220.3 calories, 10.8 g fat, 1.5 g saturated fat, 30 mg cholesterol, 15.3 g protein, 18.4 g carbohydrates, 4.4 g fiber, 720 mg sodium

Carob and Psyllium Shake
Serves 1

1 cup unsweetened vanilla soymilk
1 scoop (24.3 grams) vanilla whey protein powder
1 tablespoon unsweetened carob powder
1 tablespoon psyllium seed husks
2 teaspoons flaxseed oil
1/2 teaspoon probiotic powder
3 ice cubes

Place everything in a blender, and blend until smooth.

nutrition info per serving: 289 calories, 12 g fat, 2 g saturated fat, 15 mg cholesterol, 24 g protein, 25 g carbohydrates, 6 g fiber, 123 mg sodium

Vegetable Chicken Soup
Serves 4

1 tablespoon olive oil
1 medium onion, chopped
1 pound skinless and boneless chicken breasts, cut into bite-size pieces
6 ounces green beans, cut into bite-size pieces
1 cup chopped celery
1 zucchini, sliced
1 tablespoon fresh basil, chopped
1/2 of a 14.5-ounce can diced tomatoes, drained
4 cups chicken broth
1 teaspoon paprika
1 to 2 tablespoons raw honey
2 tablespoons lemon juice
2 teaspoons minced raw ginger
2 teaspoons pressed raw garlic
Salt and pepper to taste

1. In a large soup pot, heat the olive oil over medium-high heat for several minutes.

2. Add onion, and cook, stirring occasionally, until soft.

3. Add chicken, and continue to stir occasionally to brown lightly on all sides.

4. Add remaining ingredients, bring to a boil, and allow to simmer until vegetables are just tender and chicken is cooked through.

Nutrition info per serving: 209 calories, 4.7 g fat, 0.5 g saturated fat, 55 mg cholesterol, 26.8 g protein, 14.2 g carbohydrates, 2.6 g fiber, 745 mg sodium

Recipes courtesy of:

http://www.alternativemedicine.com/adrenal-burnout/adrenal-fatigue-fix

Relieving Stress and Removing Negativity

We've gone over dietary changes and the use of supplements for treatment of adrenal fatigue, but now we've come to the most important solution –removing sources of stress and negativity from your life. I know this seems easier said than done, but it is your health that we are talking about. Life is too short to waste it being miserable. Let's take a look at some things that you can do to change your environment and help relieve your symptoms.

Get adequate sleep - I cannot stress the importance of a good night's rest enough. It allows your body to recuperate from the activities of the day, and gives your mind a break. Your internal systems also go through a reboot in order to function at their highest capacity, so do yourself a favor, and grab at least seven to nine hours of restful sleep a night.

Exercise regularly – This builds strength and stamina, and allows for a natural release of "feel-good" hormones, taking the pressure off the poor adrenals for a change. However, for those who are already stressed, it is recommended that you start with gentler forms of exercise, such as walking, tai chi, or yoga (see below). You'll also be prepared for swimsuit season all year round.

Practice relaxation techniques – If you always wanted to know what the big deal was about yoga, now is a good time to find out. Yoga focuses the mind and promotes clarity of thought, which can help you with concentration and in eliminating useless mind chatter. Meditation is also a scientifically proven method of relaxation. Its benefits impact every aspect of the mind and body, and it is a great tool for reduction of stress. Hypnosis and biofeedback are also helpful.

Simplify your life – Many of us find that we have overextended ourselves with too many commitments, leaving little time for rest and self-care. Become a toddler again and re-learn the word "No". It can be a life saver, in more ways than one.

Change your surroundings – Many people find themselves stuck in a rut. This can produce stress, as humans like variety. You don't have to make major changes, unless you feel they're necessary. Sometimes, something as simple as painting or rearranging a room, or varying a routine can hel,p and the good feelings can encourage you to make bigger changes.

Work on your relationships – Start with the relationship with yourself and you'll find that most of the others will fall in line. Take time out from your day to have a meaningful conversation with someone, especially a loved one. Developing your interpersonal relationships will give you the support you need in difficult times.

Remove negativity from your life – Whether it's a dead-end job, a toxic relationship or person, or a poor self-image, get rid of it ASAP! Nothing will bring you down faster or ruin your sense of wellbeing worse than constant exposure to negativity. You don't have to endure it anymore, so leave! This is your life, and you deserve to be happy and healthy.

Don't be afraid to ask for help – It is said that the three hardest phrases to say are "I'm sorry," "I love you," and "Help me." We would probably never see another case of adrenal fatigue (or many other illnesses for that matter) if more of us would break the taboo and ask for help. It is not a sign of weakness or low self esteem. It is a sign of strength and self-respect. You don't have to go through rough times alone. Find a support group or provider that can help you make it through.

Take responsibility for your health – I mentioned earlier that adrenal fatigue was not a recognized diagnosis in traditional medicine. That does not make what you are experiencing any less real. You know better than anyone when your body is not working properly. Take steps to educate yourself, and find a provider who will work with you to find the problem and come up with a solution that well put you on the road to recovery. Remember the healing process begins with you.

Conclusion

Thank you again for purchasing this book!

I hope it was valuable to you not only as a sufferer of adrenal fatigue, but also to help to prevent its occurrence in the first place.

The next step is to educate yourself by reading more material concerning adrenal fatigue. Understanding and knowledge are the best medicine!

Finally, if you enjoyed this book, please take the time to share your thoughts and post a review on Amazon. It'd be greatly appreciated!

Thank you and good luck!

Christine Weil

Please leave a review and let us know what you liked about this book by going to

https://www.amazon.com/gp/css/order-history

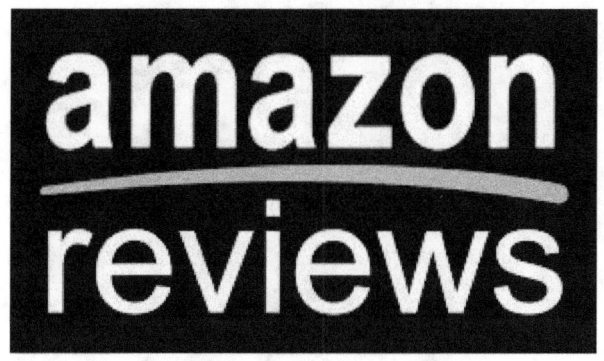

then click on Orders.

Check out the other books in the Natural Health & Natural Cures Series

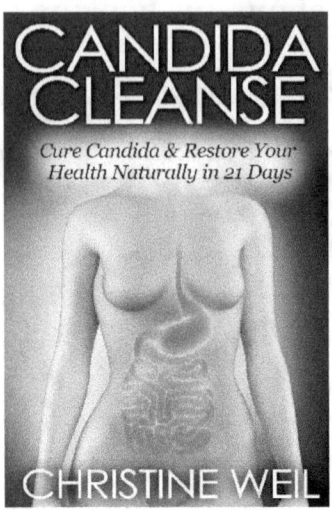

http://www.amazon.com/dp/B00IIRQH9K

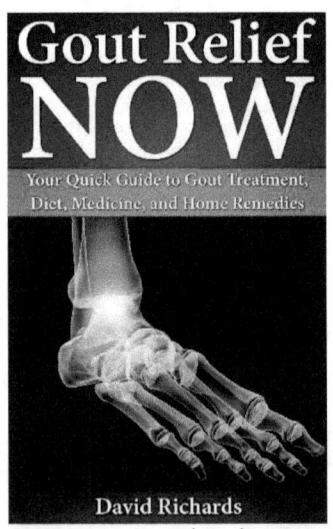

http://www.amazon.com/dp/B00HHGRBBQ

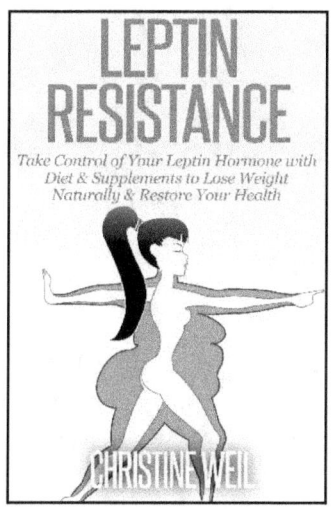

http://www.amazon.com/dp/B00J8UNBWW

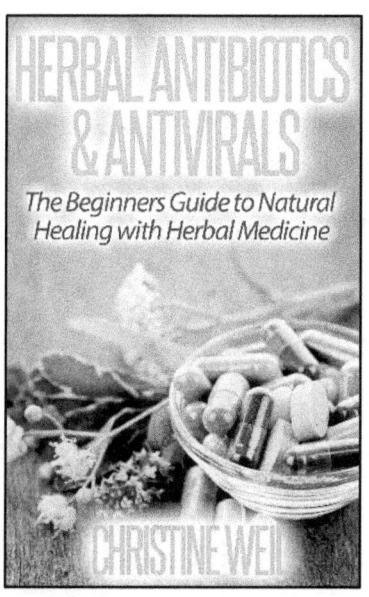

https://www.amazon.com/dp/B00J2F1QDO

Helpful Links:

http://www.alternativemedicine.com/adrenal-burnout/adrenal-fatigue-fix

http://www.drnorthrup.com/womenshealth/healthcenter/topic_details.php?topic_id=94

http://www.adrenalfatigue.org/what-is-adrenal-fatigue

http://robbwolf.com/2012/04/09/real-deal-adrenal-fatigue/

www.ingramcontent.com/pod-product-compliance
Lightning Source LLC
Chambersburg PA
CBHW071327310526
45789CB00016B/1755